Clinical Record
for
Post Basic BSc Nursing Course

Clinical Record for Post Basic BSc Nursing Course

Third Edition

C Manivannan MSc (N) MSc (Psy) MPhil (Psy) PhD (N)

Principal

Head of Department of Child Health Nursing

Sri Bharani College of Nursing

Salem, Tamil Nadu, India

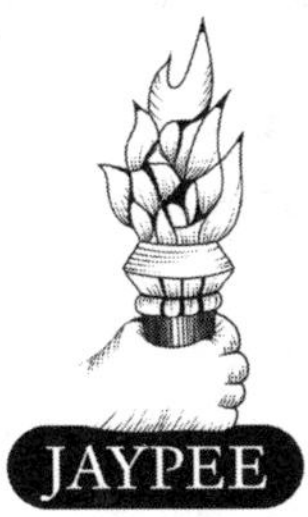

JAYPEE BROTHERS MEDICAL PUBLISHERS

The Health Sciences Publisher

New Delhi | London

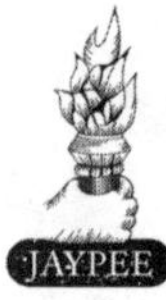

Jaypee Brothers Medical Publishers (P) Ltd

Headquarters
EMCA House
23/23-B, Ansari Road, Daryaganj
New Delhi - 110 002, India
Landline: +91-11-23272143, +91-11-23272703
+91-11-23282021, +91-11-23245672
E-mail: jaypee@jaypeebrothers.com

Corporate Office
4838/24, Ansari Road, Daryaganj
New Delhi - 110 002, India
Phone: +91-11-43574357
Fax: +91-11-43574314
E-mail: jaypee@jaypeebrothers.com

Overseas Office
J.P. Medical Ltd
83 Victoria Street, London
SW1H 0HW (UK)
Phone: +44 20 3170 8910
E-mail: info@jpmedpub.com

EU GPSR Authorised Representative
Logos Europe, 9 rue Nicolas Poussin
17000, La Rochelle, France
Phone: +33 (0) 6 67 93 73 78
E-mail: contact@logoseurope.eu

Website: www.jaypeebrothers.com
Website: www.jaypeedigital.com

Inquiries for bulk sales may be solicited at: jaypee@jaypeebrothers.com

Clinical Record for Post Basic BSc Nursing Course

First Edition: 2011

Second Edition: 2014

Third Edition: 2020, **Reprint:** 2025, **2026**

ISBN: 978-93-89188-57-8

Printed at: Samrat Offset Pvt. Ltd.

CLINICAL RECORD FOR POST BASIC BSc NURSING COURSE

PHOTOGRAPH

Name of the Institute : ....

Name of the Student : ....
(IN BLOCK LETTERS)

Father's Name : ....

Date of Birth : ....

Batch : ....

Date of Joining : ....

Date of Course Completion : ....

Registration Number : ....

Permanent Address : ....
....

Signature of the Student : ....

Date : ....

Identification Marks : 1.
2.

Name and signature of Class Coordinator	**Name and signature of Clinical Coordinator**	**Name and signature of Principal**
Date:	Date:	Date:

College seal

INSTRUCTIONS FOR USING CLINICAL RECORD

1. Procedures must be signed by the faculty.
2. Classroom procedures may be set up either in the ward (or) in the classroom.
3. Classroom procedures should not exceed 20% of the total number of procedure each year.
4. Total number of procedures for each year must be completed two weeks prior to university examination. If the required procedures are not completed by the time, the student will not be allowed to appear for the written examination.
5. Monthly records for evaluating the student's clinical performance should be kept and the average percentage should be recorded every year.

AVERAGE PERCENTAGE OF MARKS

Year	Percentage of marks	Signature of the principal
First year		
Second year		

First Year

Sl. No.	Subjects	Theory		Practical	
		Prescribed hours	Allotted hours	Prescribed hours	Allotted hours
1.	Nursing Foundation	45		–	
2.	Nutrition and Dietetics	60		15	
3.	Biochemistry and Biophysics	60		–	
4.	Psychology	60		15	
5.	Microbiology	60		30	
6.	Maternal Nursing	60		240	
7.	Child Health Nursing	60		240	
8.	Medical Surgical Nursing	60		270	
9.	English	60		-	
Total		525		810	

Name and signature of Class Coordinator

Date:

Name and signature of Clinical Coordinator

Date:

Name and signature of Principal

Date:

Second Year

Sl. No.	Subjects	Theory		Practical	
		Prescribed hours	Allotted hours	Prescribed hours	Allotted hours
1.	Sociology	60		–	
2.	Community Health Nursing	60		240	
3.	Mental Health Nursing	60		240	
4.	Introduction to Nursing Education	60		75	
5.	Introduction to Nursing Administration	60		180	
6.	Introduction to Nursing Research and statistics	45		120	
Total		345		855	

Name and signature of Class Coordinator

Date:

Name and signature of Clinical Coordinator

Date:

Name and signature of Principal

Date:

Health Record of Student

I. BASE LINE INFORMATION

Name	
Sex	
Date of Birth	
Address	
Phone number	
Local Guardian Name and Address	
Date of Admission	
Batch	
Height in cm	
Weight in kg	
Blood Group	
Rh	

II. FAMILY HEALTH RECORD

III. PERSONAL HEALTH RECORD

1. Illness During Childhood (0–12 years)	
2. Subsequent Illness (After 12 years)	
3. Physical Disability (If Any)	
4. Allergy to: (Specify) [Drug, Food, Cosmetics, Dust etc]	
5. If Female Menstrual Period	
a. Age at Menarche	
b. Frequency	
c. Duration	
d. Pain during Cycle	
e. Treatment Taken for Dysmenorrhea	
6. Obstetrical history (if married)	
7. Any Other	

IV. VACCINATION

Type	Date							Remarks
Hep B								
TT								
Cholera								
Typhoid								
BCG								
Others								

V. MEDICAL EXAMINATION (ANNUAL)

Health Status	First Year	Second Year
General Appearance		
Cardio-vascular system— Heart Sound, Pulse, Blood Pressure		
Respiratory System—Resp/mt		
Musculoskeletal System		
Gastrointestinal System		
Nervous System		
Genitourinary System		
Endocrinology		
ENT		
Eye (Acquity)		
Skin		
Dentition		
Remarks		

VI. LABORATORY FINDINGS (AS REQUIRED)

Investigation	Date	Result	Date	Result
Blood				
Hemoglobin				
X-ray				
Urine				
Routine				
Stools				
Ova/cyst				
Any others				

Date: Doctor's name:

VII. MONTHLY WEIGHT RECORD

Wt in kg	June	July	August	September	October	November	December	January	February	March	April	May
First Year												
Second Year												

VIII. MENSTRUAL HISTORY

LMP	June	July	August	September	October	November	December	January	February	March	April	May
First Year												
Second Year												

IX. (a) SUMMARY OF OUTPATIENT TREATMENT

Date	Diagnosis	Investigations/ Result	Treatment	Sick leave recommendation		Total days
				From	To	

Date: Signature of Incharge

(b) SUMMARY OF INPATIENT TREATMENT

Date	Diagnosis	Investigation/ Results	Treatment	Sick leave recommendation		Total days
				From	To	

Signature of the Class Coordinator

Signature of the Principal

MEDICAL SURGICAL NURSING

Sl. No.	Nursing procedure	Date		Signature
		Ward	Classroom	
1.	**Care Study**			
	a.			
	b.			
	c.			
2.	**Care Plans**			
	a.			
	b.			
	c.			
	d.			
	e.			
3.	**Clinical Presentation**			
	a.			
	b.			
	Health Education			
	c. Individual			
	d. Group			
4.	**Drug Presentation**			
	a.			
	b.			

Sl. No.	Nursing procedure	Date		Signature
		Ward	Classroom	
5.	**Operating Room Procedure**			
	a.			
	b.			
	c.			
	d.			
6.	**Observing for Surgeries** ***Major Operation***			
	a.			
	b.			
	c.			
	d.			
	Minor Surgeries			
	a.			
	b.			
	c.			
	d.			
7.	**Tray Setup in Surgeries**			
	A. Abdominal Surgeries a.			
	b.			

Sl. No.	Nursing procedure	Date		Signature
		Ward	Classroom	
	B. Rectal/Vaginal Surgeries			
	a.			
	b.			
	C. Orthopedic Surgeries			
	a.			
	D. Ear, Nose and Throat Surgeries			
	a.			
	b.			
	c.			
8.	**Advanced Nursing Procedures**			
9.	**Vital Signs**			
	A. Temperature			
	a. Oral			
	b. Rectal			
	c. Axilla			
	B. Pulse			
	C. Respiration			
	D. Blood Pressure			
	E. Pain			

Sl. No.	Nursing procedure	Date		Signature
		Ward	Classroom	
10.	**Assisting Special Diagnostic/Therapeutic Measures**			
	a. Abdominal Paracentesis			
	b. Thoracentesis			
	c. Pleural Tapping			
	d. Lumbar Puncture			
	e. Intracranial Pressure (ICP) Monitoring			
	f. Plaster of Paris Application			
	g. Skin/skeletal Traction			
	h. Intercostal Infusion			
	i. Intravenous Infusion			
	j. Blood Transfusion			
	k. Exchange Transfusion			
	l. Invasive/Non-invasive Hemodynamics			
11.	**Nutritional Needs/Measures**			
	A. Preparation of Fluid Diet			
	B. Maintenance of Intake–Output			
	C. Feeding the Helpless Patient Orally			
	D. Therapeutic Menu for different Patient			
	a. Diabetic Diet			
	b. Hypertensive Diet			
	c. Renal Diet			

Sl. No.	Nursing procedure	Date		Signature
		Ward	Classroom	
	E. Assisting Patients for:			
	a. Enteral			
	b. Parenteral Nutrition			
	c. Total Parenteral Nutrition			
12.	**Diagnostic Procedure/Collection of Samples**			
	A. Blood			
	a. Routine			
	b. Culture			
	B. Urine			
	a. Routine			
	b. 24 hours			
	c. Culture			
	C. Stool/Feces			
	a. Routine			
	b. Culture			
	D. Cerebrospinal Fluid (CSF)			
	a. Sugar			
	b. Albumin			
	c. CSF Smear			
	E. Sputum			
	F. Throat Swab			
	G. Others			

Sl. No.	Nursing procedure	Date		Signature
		Ward	Classroom	
13.	**Therapeutic Measures**			
	A. Oxygen Inhalation			
	B. Hot Application			
	a. Hot Water Bag			
	b. Infrared/Ultraviolet Lamp			
	C. Cold Application			
	a. Cold Compress			
	b. Ice Cap			
	c. Cold/Tepid Sponge			
14.	**Administering Oral Medication**			
15.	**Administering Injection**			
	A. Intramuscular			
	B. Intravenous			
	C. Intradermal			
	D. Hypodermic/Insulin			
16.	**Surgical Dressing**			
17.	**Surgical Soak**			
	Fomentation			

Sl. No.	Nursing procedure	Date		Signature
		Ward	Classroom	
18.	**Therapeutic Measures**			
	a. Intravenous Infusion			
	b. Blood Transfusion			
	c. Exchange Transfusion			
19.	**Preoperative Care**			
	a. Skin Preparation			
	b. Psychological Preparation			
	c. Consent			
	d. Shifting Patient to the Operation Theater (OT)			
20.	**Postoperative Care**			
	a. Unit Preparation			
	b. Immediate Postoperative Care			
	c. Maintain Recovery Room			
	d. Postoperative Exercise			
21.	**Neurological and Neurosurgical Condition**			
	a. Neurological Assessment			
	b. Assess Glasgow Coma Scale			
	c. Monitor Intracranial Pressure			
	d. Physical Preparation for Neurosurgery			

Sl. No.	Nursing procedure	Date		Signature
		Ward	Classroom	
22.	**Care of Patient with:**			
	a. Head Injury			
	b. Cerebrovascular Accident (CVA)			
	c. Spinal Cord Injury			
	d. Cranial Injury			
	e. Brain Tumor			
	f. Congenital Malformation			
	g. Degenerative Disease			
	h. Unconscious Patient			
	i. Cervical Traction			
	j. Pelvic Traction			
23.	**Preparation of Patient for:**			
	a. Computed Tomography (CT)			
	b. Electroencephalogram (EEG)			
	c. Magnetic Resonance Imaging (MRI)			
	d. Planning for Activities of Daily Living (ADL) Needs			
24.	**Cardiothoracic Procedure**			
	A. Cardiothoracic Assessment			
	B. Observation of:			

Sl. No.	Nursing procedure	Date		Signature
		Ward	Classroom	
	a. Cardiac Monitoring			
	b. Cardiac Catheterization			
	c. Echocardiogram			
	d. Electrocardiogram			
	e. Stress Test			
	f. Percutaneous Transluminal Coronary Angioplasty			
	g. Bronchography			
25.	Assist for:			
	a. Collecting Blood for Cardiac Enzymes			
	b. Insertion of Intercostal Drainage			
	c. Changing of Intercostal Drainage			
	d. Pulmonary Function Test (PFT)			
	e. Bronchoscopy			
	f. Cardiopulmonary Resuscitation (CPR)			
	g. Taking Blood for Arterial Blood Gas Analysis			
	h. Thoracentesis			
	i. Perform Mantoux Test			
	j. Pacemaker			
	k. Cardiac Diet			
	l. Defibrillation			

Sl. No.	Nursing procedure	Date		Signature
		Ward	Classroom	
26.	**Administer for:**			
	a. Steam Inhalation			
	b. Nebulization			
27.	**Genitourinary Procedure**			
	a. Kidney Ureter Bladder (KUB)			
	b. Hemodialysis			
	c. Peritoneal Dialysis			
	d. Insertion of Foley's Catheter for Male/Female			
	e. Cystoscopy			
	f. Intravenous Pyelogram (IVP)			
	g. Bladder Irrigation			
28.	**Preparation for**			
	a. Renal Angiogram			
	b. Renal Biopsy			
	c. Intravenous Urogram			
	d. Renal Transplantation			
	e. Transurethral Resection of the Prostate (TURP)			
	f. Continuous Ambulatory Peritoneal Dialysis (CAPD)			
	g. Renal Diet			

Sl. No.	Nursing procedure	Date		Signature
		Ward	Classroom	
29.	**Gastrointestinal Procedure**			
	a. Assessment of GI System			
	b. Perform Wound Dressing			
	c. Care of Drainage Tube			
	d. Administer Total Parental Nutrition			
	e. Gastrostomy Feeding			
	f. Assist in Specific Diagnostic Test			
	• Venesection			
	• Endoscopy			
	• Protoscopy			
	• Barium Meal			
	• Barium Enema			
	• Cholecystography			
	• Colostomy Tube			
	• Paracentesis			
	g. Gastric Analysis			
	h. Esophageal Balloon			
	i. Sitz Bath			
	j. Surgical Soak			
	k. Care of Drainage Tube			

Sl. No.	Nursing procedure	Date		Signature
		Ward	Classroom	
30.	**Metabolic and Endocrine Function**			
	a. Assessment of Endocrine System			
	b. Glycosylated Hemoglobin			
	c. Diabetic Diet			
	d. Glucose Tolerance Test (GTT)			
	e. Insulin Pump			
	f. Thyroid Function Test			
31.	**Assessment of Musculoskeletal System**			
32.	**Care of Patient with:**			
	a. Plaster of Paris			
	b. Traction			
	c. Fracture			
	d. Amputation /Stump Care			
	e. Internal /External Fixation			
	f. Total Hip/Knee Replacement			
	g. Rehabilitation			
33.	**Sexual and Reproductive Function**			
	a. Assessment of Reproductive Function			
	b. Infertility Clinic			
	c. Breast Self-examination			
	d. Post-mastectomy Exercise			

Sl. No.	Nursing procedure	Date		Signature
		Ward	Classroom	
34.	**Eye/ENT**			
	Application of Drops/Ointment			
	a. Eye			
	b. Ear			
	c. Nose			
35.	**Assist in:**			
	a. Eye Irrigation			
	b. Ear Irrigation			
	c. Auditory Activity			
	d. Throat Swab Culture/Throat Painting			
	e. Removal of Foreign Bodies			
36	**Burns**			
	Assessment of Patient with Burns			
37.	**Assist in:**			
	a. Burn Dressing			
	b. Reconstructive Surgery			
38.	**Administration/Calculation of Fluid and Electrolytes**			
39.	**Oncology**			
	Assist in:			
	a. Radiotherapy			
	b. Chemotherapy			
	c. Biopsy			

Sl. No.	Nursing procedure	Date		Signature
		Ward	Classroom	
	d. Bone Marrow Aspiration			
	e. PAP Smear			
40.	**Central Sterile Supply Department/ CSSD Procedure**			
	a. Rubber Goods			
	b. Dressings			
	c. Gloves			
	d. Instruments			
	e. Needles			
	f. Sutures			
	g. Syringes			
	h. Glassware			
41.	**Preparation and Packing of Articles for Surgery**			
42.	**Disinfecting the Operation Theater**			
43.	**Scrubbing**			
44.	**Gowning**			
45.	**Gloving**			
46.	**Setting-up of Sterile Trolly**			

Total Number of Procedures Signed: ....

Number of Ward Procedures: ....

Number of Classroom Procedures: ....

Name and signature of Class Coordinator

Date:

Name and signature of Clinical Coordinator

Date:

Name and signature of Principal

Date:

First Year Practical Examination for Medical Surgical Nursing

Signature of Internal Examiner :

Date :

Signature of External Examiner :

Date :

First Supplementary Examination

Signature of Internal Examiner :

Date :

Signature of External Examiner :

Date :

Second Supplementary Examination

Signature of Internal Examiner :

Date :

Signature of External Examiner :

Date :

CHILD HEALTH NURSING

Sl. No.	Nursing procedure	Date		Signature
		Ward	Classroom	
1.	**Care Study**			
	a.			
	b.			
	c.			
2.	**Care Plan**			
	a.			
	b.			
	c.			
	d.			
	e.			
3.	**Clinical Presentation**			
	a.			
	b.			
	Health Education			
	c. Individual			
	d. Group			
4.	**Drug Presentation**			
	a.			
	b.			
5.	**Admission of Children**			

Sl. No.	Nursing procedure	Date		Signature
		Ward	Classroom	
6.	**History Collection**			
7.	**Physical Assessment**			
	a. Newborn			
	b. Infant			
	c. Sick child			
8.	**Assessment of Growth and Development**			
9.	**Anthropometric Measurement**			
10.	**Assessment of Degree of Dehydration**			
11.	**Vital Signs**			
	A. Temperature			
	a. Oral			
	b. Rectal			
	c. Axilla			
	B. Pulse			
	C. Respiration			
	D. Blood Pressure			
12.	**Restraint of Children**			
	a. Mummy			
	b. Elbow			
	c. Clove Hitch			
	d. Jacket			
	e. Mitten			

Sl. No.	Nursing procedure	Date		Signature
		Ward	Classroom	
13.	**Nutritional Needs**			
	a. Breastfeeding			
	b. Artificial Feeding			
	c. Nasogastric Feeding			
	Planning Special Diet for:			
	a. Nephrotic Syndrome			
	b. Protein Energy Malnutrition			
	c. Juvenile Diabetes Mellitus			
	d. Balanced Diet/Preparation for Oral Rehydration Solution (ORS)			
14.	**Enema**			
15.	**Administration of:**			
	a. Eye Drops			
	b. Ear Drops			
	c. Nasal Drops			
	d. Steam Inhalation			
	e. Nebulization			
	f. Oxygen			
	g. Oral Medication			
	h. Intramuscular Injection			
	i. Intravenous Injection			
	j. Intradermal/Subcutaneous Injection			
16.	**Colostomy Irrigation**			

Sl. No.	Nursing procedure	Date		Signature
		Ward	Classroom	
17.	**Blood Transfusion**			
18.	**Intravenous Infusion**			
19.	**Exchange Transfusion**			
20.	**Specimen Collection**			
	a. Urine Collection for Male/Female			
	b. 24 hrs Urine Collection			
	c. Blood Collection for Neonate/Infant			
	d. Faces Collection			
	e. Cerebrospinal Fluid Collection			
	e. Throat Swab			
	g. Skin Scrapings			
21.	**Assisting in:**			
	a. Painful Procedure			
	b. Lumbar Puncture			
	c. Phototherapy			
	d. Incubator Care			
	e. Radiant Warmer			
	f. Ventilator Care			
22.	**Neonatal Resuscitation**			
23.	**Use of Splint**			
24.	**Cardiopulmonary Resuscitator for Neonate/ Infant/Toddler (CPR)**			
25.	**Preoperative Care**			

Sl. No.	Nursing procedure	Date		Signature
		Ward	Classroom	
26.	**Postoperative Care**			
27.	**Pediatric Emergency**			
	a. Asphyxia			
	b. Convulsion			
	c. Head Injury			
	d. Hemolytic Disorder			
28.	**Group Teaching**			
29.	**Field Visit**			
	a. Crèche			
	b. Anganwadi			
	c. Orphanage			
	d. Genetic Counseling			
	e. Nursery School			
	f. PHC/Subcentre			
	g. Indian Population Project Center			

Total Number of Procedures Signed: ....

Number of Ward Procedures: ....

Number of Classroom Procedures: ....

Name and signature of Class Coordinator

Date:

Name and signature of Clinical Coordinator

Date:

Name and signature of Principal

Date:

First Year Practical Examination for Child Health Nursing

Signature of Internal Examiner :

Date :

Signature of External Examiner :

Date :

First Supplementary Examination

Signature of Internal Examiner :

Date :

Signature of External Examiner :

Date :

Second Supplementary Examination

Signature of Internal Examiner :

Date :

Signature of External Examiner :

Date :

MATERNITY NURSING SKILLS

Sl. No.	Nursing procedure	Date		Signature
		Ward	Classroom	
1.	**Care Study (Antenatal/Postnatal/Gynecology)**			
	a.			
	b.			
	c.			
2.	**Care Plan (Antenatal/Postnatal/Intranatal/ Neonatal/Gynecology)**			
	a.			
	b.			
	c.			
	d.			
	e.			
3.	**Clinical Presentation**			
	a.			
	b.			
	Health Education			
	c. Individual			
	d. Group			
4.	**Drug Presentation**			
	a.			
	b.			

Sl. No.	Nursing procedure	Date		Signature
		Ward	Class room	
5.	**Visits**			
	a. Infertility Center			
	b. Antenatal Clinic			
	c. Postnatal Clinic			
	d. Immunization Clinic			
	e. Baby-Friendly Hospital Initiative			
6.	**Prenatal Care**			
	a. Prenatal Assessment			
	b. Prenatal Care			
	c. Non-stress Test			
	d. Ultrasound			
	e. Set-up of Antenatal and Postnatal Clinic			
7.	**Care of High-risk Mother in Antenatal and Postnatal**			
	a. Pre-eclampsia			
	b. Eclampsia			
	c. Placenta Previa			
	d. Abruptio Placentae			
	e. Gestational Diabetes			
	f. Rh Incompatibility			
	g. Preterm Contraction			

Sl. No.	Nursing procedure	Date		Signature
		Ward	Classroom	
	h. Cardiac Disease			
	i. Antepartum Hemorrhage (APH)			
	j. Ectopic Pregnancy			
	k. Anemia			
	l. Polyhydramnios			
	m. Hydatidiform Mole			
	n. Abortion			
	o. Postpartum Hemorrhage (PPH)			
	p. Puerperal Sepsis			
	q. Oligohydramnios			
8.	**Preparation of Patient for:**			
	A. Urine Analysis			
	a. Albumin			
	b. Glucose			
	c. Ketones			
	B. Ultrasounds			
9.	**Antenatal Palpation**			
10.	**PV Examination**			

Sl. No.	Nursing procedure	Date		Signature
		Ward	Classroom	
11.	**Administration of:**			
	a. Tetanus Toxoid, Iron, Folic Acid			
	b. Education of Mother regarding Exercise			
	• Antenatal Exercise			
	• Postnatal Exercise			
	c. Education of Mother regarding Diet			
	• Antenatal Diet			
	• Postnatal Diet			
12.	**Intranatal**			
	a. Transfer to Delivery Unit			
	b. Preparation of Mother for Delivery			
	c. Observe Signs of Progression of Labor			
	• Electronic Fetal Monitoring			
	• Observe Uterine Contraction			
	• Partogram			
	d. Management of Pain throughout Labor			
	e. Induction of Labor: Medical/Surgical			
	f. APGAR Score			
	g. Weighing Newborn			
	h. Baby Bath			

Sl. No.	Nursing procedure	Date		Signature
		Ward	Classroom	
	i. Placental Assessment			
	j. Assist Mother in Initiating Breastfeeding			
13.	**Assist in:**			
	a. Forceps Delivery			
	b. Vacuum Extraction			
	c. Breech Delivery			
	d. Multifetal Delivery/Twins			
	e. Cesarean Section			
	f. Episiotomy			
14.	**Postnatal Care**			
	a. Receive Mother from Labor Unit/ Operation Theater			
	b. Perineal Care			
	c. Postnatal Examination [BUBBLERS—Breast, Uterus, Bowel, Bladder, Lochia, Episiotomy Surgical site (Cesarean)]			
	d. Episiotomy Care			
	e. Care of High-risk Postnatal Mother			
	f. Perineal Light			
15.	**Newborn Care**			
16.	**Assessment of Preterm Baby**			

Sl. No.	Nursing procedure	Date		Signature
		Ward	Classroom	
17.	**Care of High-risk Newborn**			
	a. Baladai Feeding			
	b. Tube Feeding			
	c. Spoon Feeding			
18.	**Cord Care**			
19.	**Eye Care**			
20.	**Immunization**			
21.	**Phototherapy**			
22.	**Care of Baby in Incubator**			
23.	**Care of Baby in Radiant Warmer**			
24.	**Care of Baby on Ventilator**			
25.	**Family Welfare**			
26.	**Motivation of:**			
	a. Family for Family Planning Method			
	b. Planned Parenthood			
	c. IUD Insertion			
27.	**Assist in:**			
	a. Tubectomy			
	b. Vasectomy			

Sl. No.	Nursing procedure	Date		Signature
		Ward	Classroom	
28.	**Requirements**			
	Antenatal Examination—20			
	Postnatal Examination—20			
	Neonatal Examination—10			
	Pre Vaginal Examination—20			
	Conduct Normal Deliveries—20			
	Stitching of Episiotomy—10			
	Counseling of Family for Adopting Family Planning Method—5			
	Motivate Family for Planned Parenthood—2			
	Assisting IUD Insertion—2			
	Assist in Cesarean Section—10			

Total Number of Procedures Signed: ....

Number of Ward Procedures: ....

Number of Classroom Procedures: ....

Name and signature of Class Coordinator

Date:

Name and signature of Clinical Coordinator

Date:

Name and signature of Principal

Date:

First Year Practical Examination for Maternity Nursing Skills

Signature of Internal Examiner :

Date :

Signature of External Examiner :

Date :

First Supplementary Examination

Signature of Internal Examiner :

Date :

Signature of External Examiner :

Date :

Second Supplementary Examination

Signature of Internal Examiner :

Date :

Signature of External Examiner :

Date :

COMMUNITY HEALTH NURSING

Sl. No.	Nursing procedure	Date		Signature
		Ward	Classroom	
1.	**Care Study**			
	a.			
	b.			
	c.			
2.	**Care Plan**			
	a.			
	b.			
	c.			
3.	**Assessment of Community Resources**			
4.	**Conduct Community Survey**			
5.	**Conduct Family Survey**			
6.	**Community Report Presentation**			
7.	**Project Work**			
8.	**Assisting in:**			
	a. Antenatal Clinic			
	b. Postnatal Clinic			
	c. Family Welfare Clinic			
	d. School Health Program			

Sl. No.	Nursing procedure	Date		Signature
		Ward	Classroom	
	e. Under Five Clinic			
	f. EPI/Immunization Clinic			
	g. Health Camps			
	h. In-service Education for PHC Staff			
	i. Nutrition Education Program			
9.	**Assessment of Health**			
	a. Antenatal Care			
	b. Natal Care			
	c. Postnatal Care			
	d. Newborn			
	e. Infant			
	f. Under five			
	g. Old Age			
	h. Physically Challenged			
	i. Mentally Challenged			
10.	**Demonstration of Procedure**			
	a. Bag Technique			
	b. Hand Washing			
	c. Physical Assessment			
	d. Recording of Vital Signs			

Sl. No.	Nursing procedure	Date		Signature
		Ward	Classroom	
	e. Urine Testing			
	• Sugar			
	• Albumin			
	f. Wound Dressing			
	g. Nutritional Assessment			
	h. Administration of Medication (Oral)			
	i. Collection of Specimen			
	j. Cooking Demonstration Baby Bath			
	k. Care of Fever Patient			
	l. Oral Rehydration Therapy			
	m. Eye Irrigation			
	n. Steam Inhalation (Home)			
	o. Injection (Home)			
11.	**Health Needs**			
	a. Anthropometric Measurement			
	b. Hygienic Needs			
	c. Nutrition Needs			
	d. Elimination Needs			
	e. Emotional Needs			
	f. Spiritual Needs			

Sl. No.	Nursing procedure	Date		Signature
		Ward	Classroom	
12.	**Programs**			
	a. Community Nutrition Program			
	b. School Health Program			
13.	**Records and Reports**			
	a. Family Records			
	b. Field Visits Records			
	c. Health Education			
	d. Nutrition Education			
	e. Orientation Report			
	f. PHC Report			
14.	**Participation in National Health Program**			
15.	**Organization of Community Educating Program**			
16.	**Using Audiovisual Aids**			
	a. Flannel Graph			
	b. Flash Card			
	c. Flip Chart			
	d. Posters			
	e. Slide Projector			
	f. Puppet Show			
17.	**Health Teaching**			
	a. Individual Teaching			
	b. Group Teaching			

Sl. No.	Nursing procedure	Date		Signature
		Ward	Classroom	
18.	**Preparation of Area Map**			
	a. Urban			
	b. Rural			
19.	**Presentation of Community Visit**			
20.	**Supervision of Dais and ANM**			
21.	**Observation Visit**			
	a. Certified School			
	b. Industries			
	c. Community Mental Health Center			
	d. Subcentre/PHC/Community Health Center (CHC)			
	e. National Family Planning Association of India			
	f. Communicable Disease Hospital			
	g. National Institute of Leprosy and Tuberculosis			
	h. Voluntary Health Organization			
	i. Professional Bodies			
	• Trained Nurses Association of India (TNAI)			
	• Indian Nursing Council (INC)			
	• United Nations International Children's Emergency Fund (UNICEF)			
	• Red Cross			

Sl. No.	Nursing procedure	Date		Signature
		Ward	Classroom	
	j. Water Purification Plant			
	k. Sewage Treatment Plant			
	l. Slaughterhouse			
	m. Well Baby Clinic			

Total Number of Procedures Signed: ....

Number of Ward Procedures: ....

Number of Classroom Procedures: ....

Name and signature of Class Coordinator

Date:

Name and signature of Clinical Coordinator

Date:

Name and signature of Principal

Date:

Second Year Practical Examination for Community Health Nursing

Signature of Internal Examiner :

Date :

Signature of External Examiner :

Date :

First Supplementary Examination

Signature of Internal Examiner :

Date :

Signature of External Examiner :

Date :

Second Supplementary Examination

Signature of Internal Examiner :

Date :

Signature of External Examiner :

Date :

MENTAL HEALTH NURSING

Sl. No.	Nursing procedure	Date		Signature
		Ward	Classroom	
1.	**Care Study**			
	a.			
	b.			
	c.			
2.	**Care Plan**			
	a.			
	b.			
	c.			
	d.			
	e.			
3.	**Clinical Presentation**			
	a.			
	b.			
	Health Education			
	a. Individual			
	b. Group			
4.	**Drug Presentation**			
	a.			
	b.			

Sl. No.	Nursing procedure	Date		Signature
		Ward	Classroom	
5.	**Visits**			
	a. Child Guidance Clinic			
	b. Deaf and Dumb School			
	c. Blind/Mental Retardation School			
	d. Half-way Home			
	e. De-addiction Center			
	f. Community Mental Health Centers			
	g. Old Age Home			
6.	**Admission Procedure**			
7.	**Discharge Procedure**			
8.	**Mental Status Examination**			
9.	**Process Recording**			
10.	**Assist in:**			
	a. Convulsion Therapy			
	b. Psychotherapy			
	• Individual			
	• Group			
	• Family			
	• Community			
	c. Recreational Therapy			

Sl. No.	Nursing procedure	Date		Signature
		Ward	Classroom	
	d. Play Therapy			
	e. Drug Therapy			
	f. Social Therapy			
	g. Occupational Therapy			
	h. Behavioral Therapy			
	i. Deaddiction Therapy			
	j. Milieu Therapy			
	k. Rehabilitation Therapy			
11.	**Administration of Psychiatric Emergency Drug**			
12.	**Nursing Care of Patient with:**			
	a. Psychotic Disorder			
	b. Neurotic Disorder			
	c. Organic Disorder			
	d. Character Disorder			
	e. Substance Abuse			
	f. Conduct Disorder			
	g. Mental Retardation			
13.	**Maintain Therapeutic Communication Technique**			
14.	**Psychiatric Ward Rounds**			

Sl. No.	Nursing procedure	Date		Signature
		Ward	Classroom	
15.	**Counseling Section**			
	a. Individual			
	b. Family			
	c. Group			
	d. Psychological			
	e. Educational			
	f. Marital			

Total Number of Procedures Signed: ....

Number of Ward Procedures: ....

Number of Classroom Procedures: ....

Name and signature of Class Coordinator

Date:

Name and signature of Clinical Coordinator

Date:

Name and signature of Principal

Date:

Second Year Practical Examination for Mental Health Nursing

Signature of Internal Examiner :

Date :

Signature of External Examiner :

Date :

First Supplementary Examination

Signature of Internal Examiner :

Date :

Signature of External Examiner :

Date :

Second Supplementary Examination

Signature of Internal Examiner :

Date :

Signature of External Examiner :

Date :

INTRODUCTION TO NURSING EDUCATION

Sl. No.	Nursing procedure	Date		Signature
		Ward	Classroom	
1.	**Practice Teaching**			
	A. Classroom Teaching			
	a.			
	b.			
	c.			
	B. Clinical Teaching			
	a.			
	b.			
	c.			
2.	**Preparation of:**			
	a. Lesson Plan			
	b. Unit Plan			
	c. Course Outline			
	d. Master Rotation Plan			
	e. Clinical Rotation Plan			
	f. Audiovisual Aids			
	• Charts			
	• Posters			
	• Flash Card			

Sl. No.	Nursing procedure	Date		Signature
		Ward	Classroom	
	• Transparencies			
	• Models			
	g. Evaluation Tools			
	• Practice Teaching Evaluation			
	• Clinical Evaluation			
	• Patient Health			
	• Student Health			
	• Student Educational Performance			
3.	**Teaching Methods/Methods of Teaching**			
	a. Lecture Method			
	b. Seminar Method			
	c. Discussion Method			
	d. Demonstration Method			
	e. Laboratory Method			
	f. Project Method			
	g. Problem-solving Method			
	h. Nursing Rounds			
	i. Nursing Conference			
4.	**Observation Visit**			
	a. College of Nursing			
	b. School of Nursing			

Sl. No.	Nursing procedure	Date		Signature
		Ward	Classroom	
5.	**Student Counseling Section**			
6.	**Patient Counseling Section**			
7.	**In-service Education**			

Total Number of Procedures Signed: ....

Number of Ward Procedures: ....

Number of Class Room Procedures: ....

Name and signature of Class Coordinator

Date:

Name and signature of Clinical Coordinator

Date:

Name and signature of Principal

Date:

INTRODUCTION TO NURSING ADMINISTRATION

Sl. No.	Nursing procedure	Date		Signature
		Ward	Classroom	
1.	**Preparation of Job Description**			
	A. Hospital Staff			
	a. Nursing Superintendent			
	b. Head Nurse			
	c. Ward /ICU/OT In-charge			
	d. Staff Nurse			
	e. Nurse Aid			
	f. Class IV Workers			
	B. Educational Institution			
	a. Principal			
	b. Vice Principal			
	c. Professor (HOD)			
	d. Lecturer			
	e. Nursing Tutors			
	f. Clinical Instructor			
2.	**Supervision of:**			
	a. Staff Nurse			
	b. Student Nurses			
	c. Ward Aid			

Sl. No.	Nursing procedure	Date		Signature
		Ward	Classroom	
3.	**Ward Administration**			
	A. Cleanliness of the Ward/Hospital			
	B. Delegation of Assignment of Duties			
	a. Head Nurse			
	b. Staff Nurse			
	c. Student Nurse			
	d. Ward Workers			
	C. Preparation of Duty Roster			
	D. Maintain:			
	a. Drug Inventory			
	• General Drugs			
	• Narcotic Drugs			
	b. Ordering Drugs and Equipment			
	c. Requisition for Repair and Replacement			
	d. Equipment Inventory			
	e. Records and Reports			
	f. Management of Supplies			
	g. Student Health Record			

Sl. No.	Nursing procedure	Date		Signature
		Ward	Classroom	
4.	**Maintenance of Leadership Styles**			
5.	**Organization of:**			
	a. Health Programs			
	b. In-service Education			
	c. Clinical Presentation			
	d. Staff Development Program			
	e. Medical Camps			
	f. Conduct Nursing Conference			
6.	**Maintain Hospital Census**			
7.	**Conducting Ward Teaching**			
8.	**Preparation of Student for Demonstration in Ward**			
9.	**Patient Assignment Plan**			
10.	**Weekly Time Sheet**			
11.	**Preparation and Use of Evaluation Tools**			
	A. Hospital			
	a. Patient Care Evaluation			
	b. Student Performance Evaluation			
	c. Staff Performance Evaluation			

Sl. No.	Nursing procedure	Date		Signature
		Ward	Classroom	
	B. College			
	a. Student Teacher Evaluation			
	b. Viva Guidelines			
	c. Observation Checklist			

Total Number of Procedures Signed: ....

Number of Ward Procedures: ....

Number of Classroom Procedures: ....

Name and signature of Class Coordinator

Date:

Name and signature of Clinical Coordinator

Date:

Name and signature of Principal

Date: